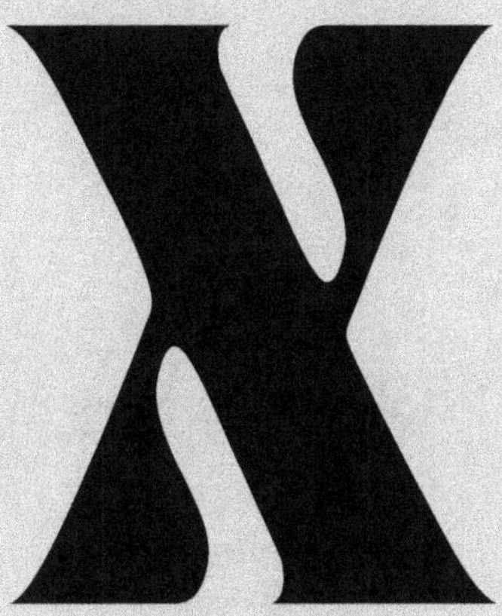

FITNESS
BOOTCAMP

In loving memory of

Mike Mentzer
(1951 - 2001)

May his fascinating studies and vast knowledge in the
field of bodybuilding live and be passed on by us

Table of content

Table of content

Understanding Fitness

Introduction:

In this chapter, we will explore the concept of fitness and its importance in our lives. By understanding the components of fitness and the benefits it offers, you will be empowered to unlock your full potential.

1.1: Defining fitness

Fitness can be defined as the ability to perform physical activities efficiently and effectively. It goes beyond just having a muscular physique. Fitness encompasses various aspects such as cardiovascular endurance, muscular strength and endurance, flexibility, and body composition.

Achieving fitness requires a holistic approach that includes regular exercise, proper nutrition, adequate rest, and a positive mindset. It is not just about looking good but also feeling good and being capable of handling the physical demands of daily life.

Fitness is a lifelong journey, and it is important to set realistic goals and work towards them gradually. It is not a quick fix or temporary solution but rather a lifestyle choice that can lead to long-term health and well-being.

1.2: The components of fitness

Fitness is not limited to just one aspect but comprises several components that contribute to overall physical well-being. As mentioned, these components include cardiovascular endurance, muscular strength and endurance, flexibility, and body composition.

Cardiovascular endurance refers to the ability of the heart, lungs, and blood vessels to deliver oxygen and nutrients to the muscles during prolonged physical activity. It can be improved through activities such as running, cycling, swimming, and aerobics.

Muscular strength and endurance are essential for performing daily tasks and preventing injuries. Strength refers to the maximum force a muscle or muscle group can exert, while endurance is the ability to sustain muscle contractions over a period of time. Resistance training exercises like weightlifting and bodyweight exercises help improve both strength and endurance.

1.3: The benefits of being fit

Being fit offers numerous benefits that extend beyond physical health. Regular exercise and a healthy lifestyle can improve mental health, boost self-confidence, enhance cognitive function, reduce the risk of chronic diseases, increase longevity, and improve overall quality of life.

Physical fitness can also improve immune function, promote better sleep, increase energy levels, and enhance mood and emotional well-being. It can help manage stress and anxiety, leading to a more balanced and fulfilling life.

Additionally, being fit allows you to engage in activities you enjoy and participate in sports or recreational pursuits without limitations. It enables you to maintain independence and perform daily tasks with ease, contributing to a higher level of functional fitness.

Importance of Fitness in Life

Introduction:

In this chapter, we will explore the importance of fitness in life and how it can positively impact your overall well-being. As said before, by incorporating fitness into your daily routine, you can enhance your physical health, improve your mental clarity, and boost your self-confidence. So let's dive in!

2.1: Enhancing overall health and well-being

Fitness plays a crucial role in enhancing your overall health and well-being. Regular physical activity helps to strengthen your immune system, reduce the risk of chronic diseases, and improve cardiovascular health. By engaging in activities such as cardio exercises, strength training, and flexibility training, you can achieve a healthier body composition, increase bone density, and lower blood pressure levels. Additionally, regular exercise aids in improving digestion, promoting better sleep, and boosting energy levels, allowing you to live a more vibrant and fulfilling life.

Furthermore, fitness is not just limited to physical health. It also has a profound impact on your mental well-being. When you exercise, your brain releases endorphins, which are chemicals that act as natural mood lifters. These endorphins help to reduce stress, anxiety, and symptoms of depression. Regular physical activity also promotes better cognitive function, memory retention, and overall mental clarity. By prioritizing fitness in your life, you can experience improved mental health and a greater sense of well-being.

Incorporating fitness into your daily routine has numerous benefits for your overall health and well-being. By taking care of your physical and mental health, you can lead a happier and more fulfilling life.

2.2: Improving mental clarity and focus

In today's fast-paced world, maintaining mental clarity and focus is essential for success. Engaging in regular physical activity has been shown to improve cognitive function and enhance mental clarity. When you exercise, your brain receives increased blood flow and oxygen, leading to improved cognitive abilities such as memory, attention span, and problem-solving skills. Studies have also shown that regular exercise can reduce the risk of cognitive decline and age-related mental disorders, such as dementia.

Regular physical activity also helps to reduce stress levels and improve your ability to concentrate. When you exercise, your body releases stress-fighting hormones, such as norepinephrine, which helps to alleviate anxiety and improve focus. By incorporating fitness into your daily routine, you can experience improved mental clarity, increased productivity, and enhanced overall cognitive function.

Whether you engage in aerobic exercises, yoga, or strength training, regular physical activity can significantly improve your mental clarity and focus. By prioritizing fitness in your life, you can optimize your cognitive abilities and achieve greater success in all areas of your life.

2.3: Boosting self-confidence and self-esteem

Fitness plays a vital role in boosting self-confidence and self-esteem. When you engage in regular physical activity and witness improvements in your strength, endurance, and overall fitness level, it provides a sense of accomplishment and boosts your self-confidence. Setting and achieving fitness goals can help you develop discipline, perseverance, and a positive mindset that can be applied to other areas of your life.

Physical fitness also improves your body image and self-esteem. Regular exercise helps to tone your muscles, improve posture, and enhance your overall physical appearance. By taking care of your body and achieving your desired fitness goals, you can feel more confident in your own skin and develop a positive body image.

Losing Fat and Gaining Muscle with HIT

Introduction:

In this chapter, we will explore the effective strategies for losing fat and gaining muscle through high-intensity training (HIT). Understanding the principles of high-intensity training is crucial for achieving your fitness goals. By incorporating these strategies into your workout routine, you will be able to transform your body and unlock your full potential.

3.1: Understanding the Principles of High-Intensity Training

High-intensity training, also known as HIT, is a form of exercise that involves short bursts of intense activity followed by brief periods of rest. This type of training is highly effective for fat loss and muscle building because it allows you to maximize your workout time and increase your overall calorie burn.

One of the key principles of high-intensity training is the concept of intensity. During a high-intensity workout, you should aim to push yourself to your maximum effort level. This can be achieved by performing exercises that challenge your cardiovascular system and engage multiple muscle groups simultaneously.

Another important principle of high-intensity training is the concept of progression. As you become more fit and your body adapts to the workouts, it's essential to continually challenge yourself by increasing the intensity or duration of your exercises. This will ensure that you continue to make progress and avoid hitting a plateau.

3.2: Effective Strategies for Fat Loss

When it comes to losing fat, high-intensity training can be a game-changer. By incorporating HIT workouts into your routine, you can increase your metabolism, burn more calories, and shed excess body fat. Here are some effective strategies for fat loss through high-intensity training:

Interval Training:

Interval training involves alternating between periods of high-intensity exercise and periods of low-intensity or rest. This type of training has been shown to be highly effective for fat loss and can be done with various exercises such as running, cycling, or bodyweight exercises.

Compound Movements:

Incorporating compound exercises into your high-intensity workouts can help you burn more calories and engage multiple muscle groups simultaneously. Compound movements, such as squats, deadlifts, and bench press, are highly effective for fat loss and muscle building.

Circuit Training:

Circuit training involves performing a series of exercises back to back with little to no rest in between. This type of training keeps your heart rate elevated throughout the workout, leading to increased calorie burn and fat loss. Designing a circuit that includes both cardiovascular and strength exercises can maximize your results.

3.3: Building Lean Muscle Mass

In addition to fat loss, high-intensity training can also help you build lean muscle mass. By incorporating certain techniques and strategies, you can maximize muscle growth and achieve a more toned and defined physique. Here are some effective strategies for building lean muscle mass through high-intensity training:

Progressive Overload:

To build muscle, you need to continually challenge your muscles by increasing the resistance or difficulty of your exercises. Incorporating progressive overload into your high-intensity workouts, such as increasing the weight you lift or the number of repetitions you perform, can stimulate muscle growth and development.

Time Under Tension:

Performing exercises with a slower tempo and focusing on the eccentric (lowering) phase of the movement can increase the time under tension for your muscles. This prolonged muscle contraction can stimulate muscle growth and enhance muscle definition.

Proper Nutrition:

Building lean muscle mass requires proper nutrition to support muscle repair and growth. Ensure you consume enough protein, carbohydrates, and healthy fats to fuel your workouts and promote muscle recovery. Additionally, staying adequately hydrated is essential for optimal muscle function and growth.

Final Note

By incorporating these strategies into your high-intensity training routine, you will be able to effectively lose fat and build lean muscle mass. Remember to listen to your body, gradually increase the intensity of your workouts, and prioritize proper nutrition and recovery for optimal results.

Muscle Hypertrophy through HIT

Introduction:

Muscle hypertrophy, or the growth of muscle fibers, is a goal for many individuals engaged in strength training and bodybuilding. Understanding the mechanisms behind muscle growth is essential for optimizing hypertrophy. In this chapter, we will explore the various factors that contribute to muscle growth and how high-intensity training can be utilized to achieve maximum hypertrophy. Additionally, we will discuss nutrition strategies that support muscle growth and provide the necessary fuel for intense training sessions.

4.1: Understanding Muscle Growth Mechanisms

Before diving into the specifics of high-intensity training for muscle hypertrophy, it is crucial to understand the mechanisms that drive muscle growth. There are two primary mechanisms involved in muscle hypertrophy: mechanical tension and metabolic stress.

Mechanical tension refers to the stress placed on the muscle fibers during resistance training. When muscles are subjected to high levels of mechanical tension, it triggers a series of cellular responses that ultimately lead to muscle growth. These responses include the activation of satellite cells, increased protein synthesis, and the addition of contractile proteins.

Metabolic stress, on the other hand, is the accumulation of metabolic byproducts, such as lactate and hydrogen ions, within the muscle during intense exercise. This metabolic stress stimulates the release of anabolic hormones, including growth hormone and insulin-like growth factor 1 (IGF-1), which promote muscle protein synthesis and hypertrophy.

4.2: Optimizing Hypertrophy through Training Techniques

High-intensity training is a popular approach for maximizing muscle hypertrophy. This training technique involves performing exercises with heavy loads and pushing the muscles to their limits. By doing so, it creates the necessary mechanical tension and metabolic stress to stimulate muscle growth.

One effective training technique for hypertrophy as mentioned in previous chapters, is progressive overload. This involves gradually increasing the resistance or intensity of the exercises over time. By continually challenging the muscles with heavier weights or more difficult movements, it forces them to adapt and grow stronger.

Another important aspect of high-intensity training for hypertrophy is incorporating compound exercises. Compound exercises engage multiple muscle groups simultaneously and allow for greater overall muscle recruitment. Once again, exercises such as squats, deadlifts, and bench presses are excellent choices for promoting muscle hypertrophy.

4.3: Nutrition Strategies for Muscle Growth

In addition to training techniques, proper nutrition is crucial for supporting muscle growth. To optimize muscle hypertrophy, it is essential to consume an adequate amount of protein. Protein provides the building blocks necessary for muscle repair and growth. It is said, that you should aim to consume around 1.6 - 2.2 grams of protein per kilogram of body weight per day.

Carbohydrates are also important for fueling high-intensity training sessions. When engaging in intense exercise, the body primarily relies on carbohydrates for energy. Consuming an adequate amount of carbohydrates, especially around training sessions, ensures that your muscles have enough glycogen stores to perform at their best.

Lastly, don't overlook the importance of adequate hydration. Staying hydrated is essential for optimal muscle function and recovery. Aim to drink at least 8 cups (64 ounces) of water per day, and increase your intake during intense training sessions or hot weather.

Final Note

By understanding the mechanisms of muscle growth, utilizing high-intensity training techniques, and implementing proper nutrition strategies, you can optimize muscle hypertrophy. Remember to always prioritize proper form and technique during your workouts to minimize the risk of injury. Consistency and dedication are key when it comes to achieving your muscle growth goals. Keep pushing yourself, and you will see the results you desire.

Maintaining Muscle Mass

Introduction:

In order to maintain muscle mass, it is important to understand the role of resistance training, implement strategies for preventing muscle loss, and stay motivated and consistent with your fitness routine. This chapter will provide valuable information and tips on how to effectively maintain muscle mass.

5.1: The Role of Resistance Training

Resistance training plays a crucial role in maintaining muscle mass. When you engage in resistance exercises such as weightlifting or bodyweight exercises, it stimulates your muscles to adapt and grow stronger. This helps prevent muscle loss as you age or during periods of inactivity.

Additionally, resistance training can improve your overall body composition by increasing muscle mass and reducing body fat. This not only enhances your physical appearance but also improves your metabolism and overall health.

5.2: Strategies for Preventing Muscle Loss

To effectively prevent muscle loss, it is important to implement certain strategies into your fitness routine. One key strategy is to prioritize protein intake. Protein is the building block of muscles, and consuming an adequate amount of protein can help maintain muscle mass.

In addition to protein intake, resistance training should be a regular part of your routine. Aim to engage in resistance exercises at least two to three times per week, targeting all major muscle groups. This will help preserve and build muscle mass.

Another important strategy is to include regular cardiovascular exercise. While resistance training is crucial for maintaining muscle mass, cardiovascular exercise helps improve overall cardiovascular health and can assist in maintaining a healthy body weight, which is beneficial for muscle maintenance.

5.3: Tips for Staying Motivated and Consistent

Maintaining muscle mass requires consistency and motivation. Here are some tips to help you stay on track:

Set realistic goals:

Set achievable goals that align with your fitness level and lifestyle. This will help you stay motivated and focused.

Find a workout buddy:

Working out with a friend or joining group classes can provide accountability and motivation.

Track your progress:

Keep a record of your workouts, including weights lifted and exercises performed. Seeing progress can be highly motivating.

Mix up your routine:

Trying new exercises or workout routines can keep things interesting and prevent boredom.

Reward yourself:

Set up a reward system for achieving your fitness goals, such as treating yourself to a massage or a new workout outfit.

Stay positive and be patient:

Building and maintaining muscle mass takes time and consistency. Stay positive, believe in yourself, and be patient with the process.

Final Note

By following these strategies and tips, you can effectively maintain muscle mass and enjoy the numerous benefits of a strong and healthy body.

The Importance of Muscle Recovery

Introduction:

In this chapter, we will delve into the important role that rest and recovery play in optimizing your muscle growth and overall fitness. Understanding the importance of muscle recovery is essential for anyone looking to achieve their fitness goals and prevent overtraining and injuries. In this chapter, we will explore various strategies for optimizing recovery and preventing overtraining and injuries.

6.1: Understanding the Role of Rest and Recovery

Rest and recovery are often overlooked aspects of fitness training, but they are just as important as the actual workouts themselves. When you engage in intense physical activity or strength training exercises, your muscles undergo stress and micro-tears. It is during the recovery phase that your muscles repair and rebuild, ultimately leading to increased strength and muscle growth.

Rest and recovery also play a crucial role in preventing burnout and overtraining. When you continuously push your body without allowing it sufficient time to recover, you can experience decreased performance, increased risk of injuries, and even mental fatigue. Taking the time to rest and recover allows your body to regain its energy and function optimally.

Furthermore, rest and recovery are essential for maintaining a healthy hormonal balance. Intense workouts can put stress on your endocrine system, affecting hormone levels such as cortisol, testosterone, and growth hormone. Adequate rest and recovery help restore hormonal balance, which is crucial for optimal muscle growth and overall well-being.

6.2: Strategies for Optimizing Recovery

There are several strategies you can implement to optimize your muscle recovery and enhance your overall fitness progress. One of the most important aspects is ensuring you get enough sleep. During sleep, your body goes through various restorative processes, including muscle repair and growth. Aim for 7 - 9 hours of quality sleep each night to support optimal recovery.

Another key strategy is proper nutrition. Consuming a balanced diet that includes sufficient protein, carbohydrates, and healthy fats is crucial for muscle recovery. Protein, in particular, is essential for muscle repair and growth. Be sure to include lean sources of protein in your meals, such as chicken, fish, tofu, or legumes.

Active recovery techniques can also be beneficial in promoting muscle recovery. Engaging in low-intensity exercises, such as walking or yoga, on your rest days can help increase blood flow to your muscles, aiding in their recovery. Additionally, incorporating foam rolling, stretching, or massage therapy into your routine can help alleviate muscle soreness and improve flexibility.

6.3: Preventing Overtraining and Injuries

Overtraining can have detrimental effects on your progress and overall well-being. It occurs when you consistently push your body beyond its capacity to recover, leading to decreased performance, chronic fatigue, and an increased risk of injuries. To prevent overtraining, it's important to listen to your body and recognize the signs of overtraining, such as persistent muscle soreness, decreased motivation, and difficulty sleeping.

One effective way to prevent overtraining is to incorporate rest days into your training schedule. These rest days allow your body to recover and adapt to the stress of exercise. Additionally, incorporating periodization into your training program can help prevent overtraining. Periodization involves varying the intensity and volume of your workouts over specific periods to allow for adequate recovery and prevent stagnation.

Proper warm-up and cool-down routines are also crucial in preventing injuries. Taking the time to warm up your muscles before exercise helps increase blood flow and flexibility, reducing the risk of strains or sprains. Similarly, cooling down after a workout helps your body gradually transition to a resting state, reducing the chance of post-exercise muscle soreness and stiffness.

Final Note

In conclusion, understanding the importance of muscle recovery is essential for anyone looking to optimize their fitness progress and prevent overtraining and injuries. Rest and recovery play a vital role in muscle repair, hormonal balance, and overall well-being. By implementing strategies such as sufficient sleep, proper nutrition, and active recovery techniques, you can enhance your body's recovery process and achieve your fitness goals more effectively.

The Significance of Nutrition

Introduction:

In order to achieve optimal results in bodybuilding, it is important to understand the significance of nutrition. Proper nutrition provides the building blocks necessary for muscle growth and repair, as well as the energy needed to fuel intense workouts. This chapter will delve into the role of macronutrients in muscle building, the importance of meal planning and timing, and the use of supplements for enhancing performance and recovery.

7.1: The Role of Macronutrients in Muscle Building

Macronutrients, consisting of protein, carbohydrates, and fats, play a vital role in muscle building. Protein is often considered the most important macronutrient for bodybuilders, as it provides the essential amino acids needed for muscle repair and growth. Carbohydrates serve as the primary fuel source for intense workouts, providing energy for optimal performance. Fats are also important, as they aid in hormone production and support overall health. Balancing and consuming these macronutrients in the right proportions is crucial for muscle building.

Protein:

Protein is composed of amino acids, which are the building blocks of muscles. Adequate protein intake is necessary to repair and build muscle tissue after intense workouts. Bodybuilders typically aim for a higher protein intake, ranging from 1.6 - 2.2 grams of protein per kilogram of body weight per day.

Carbohydrates:

Carbohydrates are the primary source of energy for the body, especially during intense workouts. Consuming carbohydrates before and after workouts helps replenish glycogen stores and provide the energy needed for optimal performance. Complex carbohydrates such as whole grains, fruits, and vegetables are preferred over simple sugars to ensure sustained energy levels

Fats:

While fats have often been demonized, they play a crucial role in bodybuilding. Fats support hormone production, aid in nutrient absorption, and provide insulation for vital organs. Including healthy fats such as avocados, nuts, and olive oil in your diet is essential for overall health and muscle building.

7.2: Meal Planning and Timing for Optimal Results

Meal planning and timing are key factors in maximizing muscle growth and recovery. Properly structured meals and timing can optimize nutrient absorption, fuel workouts, and support muscle repair. Here are some important considerations when planning your meals:

Caloric Intake:

To build muscle, you need to consume more calories than you burn. Calculating your daily caloric needs and ensuring a slight caloric surplus is essential. This surplus provides the energy and nutrients necessary for muscle growth.

Meal Frequency:

Dividing your daily caloric intake into multiple meals throughout the day can help maximize nutrient absorption and support muscle repair. Aim for around five to six meals per day, spaced evenly to maintain a consistent supply of nutrients.

Pre-Workout Nutrition:

Consuming a balanced meal or snack containing protein and carbohydrates before a workout can provide the necessary energy and nutrients for optimal performance. This meal should be consumed 1 - 3 hours before your workout to avoid discomfort during exercise.

Post-Workout Nutrition:

The post-workout meal is crucial for muscle recovery and growth. Consuming protein and carbohydrates within 30 - 60 minutes after a workout can help replenish glycogen stores, initiate muscle repair, and stimulate protein synthesis.

7.3: Supplements for Enhancing Performance and Recovery

While proper nutrition should always be the foundation of any bodybuilding regimen, supplements can offer additional benefits to enhance performance and recovery. Here are some commonly used supplements in the bodybuilding community:

Protein Supplements:

Protein supplements such as whey protein powder are popular among bodybuilders for their convenience and ability to provide a high-quality source of protein. They can be consumed pre or post-workout to support muscle repair and growth.

Creatine:

Creatine is a naturally occurring compound in the body that plays a role in energy production during intense exercise. Supplementing with creatine has been shown to increase strength, power, and muscle mass. It is typically consumed before or after workouts.

Branched-Chain Amino Acids (BCAAs):

BCAAs, consisting of leucine, isoleucine, and valine, are essential amino acids that help promote muscle protein synthesis and reduce muscle breakdown. BCAA supplements can be consumed before, during, or after workouts to support muscle recovery and growth.

Pre-Workout Supplements:

Pre-workout supplements often contain a combination of ingredients such as caffeine, beta-alanine, and nitric oxide boosters to enhance energy, focus, and performance during workouts. These supplements are typically taken 30 - 60 minutes before exercise.

Final Note

It is important to note that while supplements can be beneficial, they should not replace a well-balanced diet. They should be used as a complement to proper nutrition and training.

Powerlifting and Building Strength

Introduction:

Chapter 8 explores the principles of powerlifting and how it can help you build strength. Powerlifting is a strength sport that involves three main lifts: the squat, bench press, and deadlift. By understanding the principles of powerlifting and incorporating them into your training, you can maximize your strength gains and achieve your fitness goals. This chapter will delve into the concept of progressive overload, which is essential for building strength, and provide you with various training programs designed specifically for strength gains

8.1: Principles of Powerlifting

Powerlifting is a strength sport that focuses on three main lifts: the squat, the bench press, and the deadlift. The principles of powerlifting revolve around showcasing an athlete's maximal strength in these three specific movements. The key principles include:

Maximal Strength:

Powerlifting is about lifting the heaviest weights you can for a single repetition in each of the three lifts. It's not about speed or endurance but rather the ability to generate force against heavy resistance.

Intensity and Rest:

Powerlifting training involves periods of high-intensity lifting to build strength, combined with adequate rest and recovery to allow muscles to grow and adapt. Normally, these rest periods are longer than what hypertrophy training requires.

Focus on Strength, Not Aesthetics:

Powerlifting emphasizes functional strength over aesthetic appearance. Athletes focus on increasing their performance in the three lifts rather than achieving a particular physique.

8.2: Building Strength through Progressive Overload

Progressive overload is the key principle for building strength in powerlifting. It involves gradually increasing the demand on your muscles over time to stimulate adaptations and strength gains. This section will cover:

Increasing Training Volume:

Training volume refers to the total amount of work performed in a training session or week. To increase strength gains, gradually boost training volume by adding more sets, increasing reps, or raising weights. Explore methods like drop sets, super sets, and rest-pause sets. Vary rep ranges and alternate between high and low volume phases. Prioritize form, recovery, and gradual progression to avoid injury and burnout.

Gradually Increasing Intensity:

Intensity refers to the level of effort or weight lifted during training. Gradually intensify workouts by adding weight with progressive resistance, or using techniques like drop sets and supersets. Mix methods, prioritize form, and monitor progress. Balance intensity with rest and listen to your body to avoid injury.

Varying Training Frequency:

Training frequency refers to how often you train a specific muscle or movement. Varying training frequency is crucial to prevent plateaus and enhance strength gains. It prevents adaptation, optimizes recovery, stimulates muscle fibers, and prevents overuse injuries. Adjusting frequency also keeps workouts engaging and sustains progress over the long term.

8.3: Training Programs for Strength Gains

Effective training programs are essential for building strength in powerlifting. This section will provide you with various training programs designed specifically for strength gains:

Beginner Powerlifting Program:

This section will outline a beginner powerlifting program that focuses on building a solid foundation of strength and technique.

Focus on Technique:

Emphasize proper form and technique for the squat, bench press, and deadlift. Spend time mastering the basic movement patterns.

Build a Foundation:

Start with lighter weights to establish a foundation of strength and to prevent injury. Use compound lifts and gradually increase intensity.

Full-Body Workouts:

Incorporate full-body workouts with a balanced distribution of squat, bench press, and deadlift variations. Include accessory exercises to address weak points.

Progressive Overload:

Gradually increase weight, reps, or sets to challenge the muscles and promote strength gains. Aim for steady progress over time.

Rest and Recovery:

Allow sufficient rest between sessions to avoid burnout and support muscle recovery. Beginners may benefit from 2-3 days of training per week.

Intermediate Powerlifting Program:

Once you have developed a strong foundation, it's time to progress to an intermediate powerlifting program. This section will outline an intermediate program that emphasizes progressive overload and introduces more complex training techniques.

Periodization:

Implement structured cycles of training, such as linear or undulating periodization, to systematically vary intensity and volume for continued progress.

Specificity:

Focus on sport-specific movements and variations of the squat, bench press, and deadlift. Incorporate competition-style training to prepare for meets.

Accessory Work:

Include targeted accessory exercises to address weaknesses and imbalances. These exercises can enhance overall strength and stability.

Volume and Intensity:

Balance high-intensity weeks with higher-volume weeks to avoid plateaus. Manipulate sets, reps, and weights strategically.

Recovery Strategies:

Prioritize recovery through proper nutrition, sleep, and mobility work. Active recovery days can help manage fatigue.

Advanced Powerlifting Program:

For experienced lifters looking to take their strength to the next level, an advanced powerlifting program is important. This section will provide an overview of an advanced program that incorporates advanced training methods and periodization to maximize strength gains.

Advanced Periodization:

Utilize more complex periodization strategies like conjugate or block periodization to optimize strength, power, and peaking for competition.

Individualization:

Tailor programming to an athlete's unique strengths, weaknesses, and recovery capacity. Personalized training plans can yield better results.

Variation:

Introduce advanced variations of the main lifts and specialized exercises to target specific muscle groups and movement patterns.

Deloads and Peaking:

Incorporate planned deload weeks to manage fatigue and reduce injury risk. Implement peaking protocols leading up to competition for optimal performance.

Mind-Muscle Connection:

Emphasize mental focus and mind-muscle connection during lifts. Advanced lifters often refine technique to maximize efficiency.

Recovery Management:

Employ advanced recovery techniques such as sports massage, cryotherapy, and advanced nutritional strategies to optimize recovery.

Designing the Perfect Workout Routine

Introduction:

In this chapter, we will delve into the aspects of designing a workout routine that suits your specific goals and fitness level. By understanding how to identify your goals, create a balanced routine, and effectively schedule and organize your workouts, you will be on your way to achieving optimal results.

9.1: Identifying Your Goals and Fitness Level

Before diving into designing your workout routine, it is essential to first identify your goals and assess your current fitness level. By doing so, you can tailor your routine to meet your specific needs and avoid any potential setbacks or injuries.

Assessing Your Goals:

Start by clearly defining what you want to achieve through your workouts. Whether it is weight loss, muscle gain, improved cardiovascular fitness, or overall wellness, knowing your goals will help you select the right exercises and training methods.

Evaluating Your Fitness Level:

Understanding your current fitness level helps in determining where to start and how to progress effectively. Consider factors such as strength, endurance, flexibility, and any existing injuries or limitations. This assessment will guide you in selecting appropriate exercises and setting realistic expectations.

Seeking Professional Guidance:

If you are unsure about assessing your goals or fitness level, it is always beneficial to consult with a fitness professional who can provide expert advice and guidance. They can ensure your routine aligns with your capabilities.

9.2: Creating a Balanced and Effective Routine

Once you have a clear understanding of your goals and fitness level, it is time to create a workout routine that is both balanced and effective. This section will guide you through the key considerations and steps involved in designing a routine that maximizes your progress.

Selecting the Right Exercises:

Choose exercises that target all major muscle groups and cater to your specific goals. Include a mix of cardiovascular exercises, strength training exercises, and flexibility exercises to achieve a well-rounded routine.

Determining Frequency and Duration:

Determine how often you will work out and for how long. Consider factors such as your availability, recovery time, and the specific goals you want to achieve. It is essential to find the right balance between pushing yourself and allowing your body to rest and recover.

Planning Progression:

Gradually increase the intensity and complexity of your workouts to challenge your body and continue making progress. Implementing progressive overload techniques, such as increasing weight, repetitions, or duration, will help you avoid plateaus and continuously improve.

9.3: Tips for Scheduling and Organizing Workouts

Even with a perfectly designed workout routine, effective scheduling and organization are needed for consistency and long-term success. This section provides valuable tips to help you optimize your workout schedule and stay on track.

Prioritizing Consistency:

Consistency is key when it comes to achieving results. Set aside dedicated time for your workouts and treat them as non-negotiable appointments with yourself. Consider your daily routine, work schedule, and personal preferences to determine the best time to exercise.

Balancing Rest and Recovery:

Building rest days into your routine is just as important as the actual workouts. Give your body time to recover and repair to prevent overtraining and reduce the risk of injuries. Listen to your body and adjust your schedule accordingly.

Creating a Schedule and Tracking Progress:

Plan your workouts in advance and create a schedule that fits seamlessly into your lifestyle. Use tools such as workout planners or mobile apps to track your progress, monitor your achievements, and stay motivated. Having a visual representation of your routine can help you stay organized and motivated.

Final Note

By following the guidelines outlined in this chapter, you will be well-equipped to design the perfect workout routine that aligns with your goals, fitness level, and schedule. Remember, consistency, proper planning, and listening to your body are key to achieving the desired results and maintaining a lifelong commitment to fitness.

Conclusion

In this final chapter, we want to encourage you to take action and provide some final thoughts on the importance of fitness. Throughout this course, we have discussed various aspects of fitness transformation, from setting goals to developing a consistent exercise routine. Now, it's time to put everything into practice and unlock your full potential.

10.1: Take Action Now

It's easy to get caught up in the planning and preparation stages of your fitness journey. However, without taking action, all the knowledge and strategies you've learned will be for naught. It's important to remember that progress is made through consistent effort and dedication.

Start by setting small, achievable goals that align with your overall fitness vision. These goals could include working out three times a week, increasing your daily steps, or incorporating more vegetables into your meals. Whatever it may be, make a commitment to yourself and take the necessary steps to achieve those goals.

Additionally, surround yourself with a supportive network. Find a workout buddy or join a fitness community where you can share your progress, challenges, and triumphs. Having people who understand and support your fitness journey can make a significant difference in your motivation and accountability.

10.2: Final thoughts on the importance of fitness

Fitness isn't just about looking good or fitting into a certain dress size. It's about taking care of your body and mind, and unlocking your full potential in all areas of life. Regular exercise and healthy lifestyle choices have a profound impact on your physical and mental wellbeing.

When you prioritize fitness, you improve your cardiovascular health, strengthen your muscles, and boost your immune system. This leads to increased energy levels and overall vitality. You'll find that everyday tasks become easier, and you have more endurance to tackle physical challenges.

Beyond the physical benefits, fitness also has a positive impact on your mental health. As mentioned, exercise releases endorphins, which are natural mood boosters to helps reduce stress, anxiety, and symptoms of depression. By incorporating fitness into your routine, you'll experience improved mental clarity, enhanced focus, and better sleep.

Furthermore, fitness transformation is a journey of personal growth and self-discovery. As you overcome physical and mental barriers, you develop resilience, discipline, and confidence. These qualities extend beyond the gym and into all aspects of your life, empowering you to achieve your goals and face challenges head-on.

Remember, fitness is a lifelong commitment. It's not a quick fix or a temporary solution. It's a lifestyle that requires consistency and dedication. Embrace the journey, celebrate your progress, and continue to challenge yourself to reach new heights.

Thank you for joining us on this fitness transformation journey. We hope this course has provided you with valuable insights and practical strategies to unlock your full potential. Now, it's time to take action and start transforming your life through fitness. Good luck!

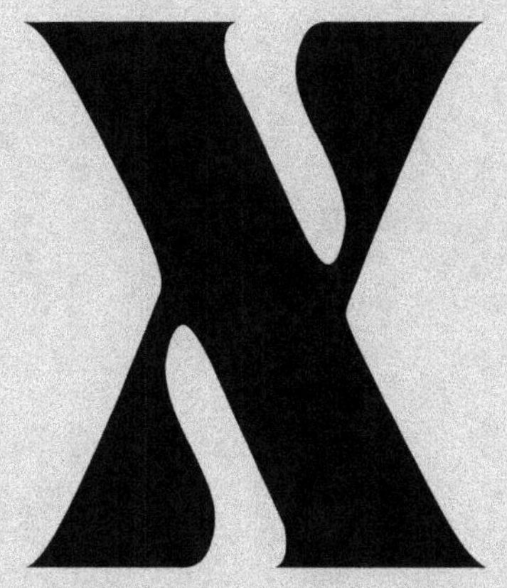